MPOX (MONKEYPOX) VIRUS:

WHY IS IT SPREADING SO QUICKLY?

Author: Raj Kishor Mahapatra

TABLE OF CONTENTS

1. Disclaimer
2. Description
3. Key Facts
4. Overview
5. Transmission
6. Signs and Symptoms
7. Diagnosis
8. Treatment and Vaccination
9. Self-care and Prevention
10. Outbreaks
11. WHO Response
12. Patient's Guide to Mpox Treatment with TPOXX (Tecovirimat)
13. Mpox Monitoring and Risk Assessment for Persons Exposed in the Community

DISCLAIMER

The information contained in this book, **"MPOX (Monkeypox) Virus: Why is it Spreading So Quickly?"** by Raj Kishor Mahapatra, is provided for general informational and educational purposes only. While the author has endeavoured to present accurate and up-to-date information based on current knowledge and research at the time of writing, this book is not intended to serve as a substitute for professional medical advice, diagnosis, or treatment.

The reader should not rely on the information contained in this book for making any health-related decisions. Always seek the advice of your physician or other qualified health providers with any questions you may have regarding a medical condition. Do not disregard professional medical advice or delay seeking it because of something you have read in this book.

The author and publisher make no representations or warranties of any kind, express or implied, regarding the completeness, accuracy, reliability, suitability, or availability of the information, products, services, or related graphics contained in this book for any purpose. Any reliance you place on such information is therefore strictly at your own risk.

In no event will the author, publisher, or any affiliated parties be liable for any loss or damage, including without limitation, indirect or consequential loss or damage, or any loss or damage whatsoever arising from loss of data or profits arising out of, or in connection with, the use of this book.

Through this book, you may be able to link to other websites that are not under the control of the author or publisher. The inclusion of any links does not necessarily imply a recommendation or endorse the views expressed within them.

Medical knowledge and practices are constantly evolving. The reader is advised to consult recent guidelines and resources for the latest information and practices regarding the management and treatment of monkeypox.

The author and publisher reserve the right to make changes to this book at any time without prior notice. Any such changes will be incorporated into updated editions of the book.

By reading this book, you agree to the terms of this disclaimer. If you do not agree to the terms of this disclaimer, you should not use this book.

DESCRIPTION

The emergence and rapid spread of the MPOX (Monkeypox) virus have raised significant concerns globally. With cases appearing in both endemic and non-endemic regions, understanding the dynamics of this virus is more crucial than ever. **"MPOX (Monkeypox) Virus: Why is it Spreading So Quickly?"** by Raj Kishor Mahapatra is an essential guide designed to provide a comprehensive understanding of this virus, its transmission, and the measures necessary to control its spread.

In this book, readers will find an in-depth exploration of the monkeypox virus, including its origins, transmission mechanisms, clinical presentation, and the current state of diagnosis and treatment. The author, Raj Kishor Mahapatra, combines his expertise in cybersecurity, writing, and health communication to present a clear and accessible resource for both healthcare professionals and the general public.

Key topics covered include:

- **Key Facts**: A quick reference to the most critical information about monkeypox, providing readers with a solid foundation of knowledge.
- **Overview**: A detailed introduction to the monkeypox virus, including its history, epidemiology, and the factors contributing to its recent spread.
- **Transmission**: Insight into how the virus spreads from animals to humans and between humans, highlighting the importance of understanding transmission pathways for effective prevention.
- **Signs and Symptoms**: A comprehensive look at the clinical

manifestations of monkeypox, helping readers identify potential cases based on symptomatology.
- **Diagnosis**: Information on the diagnostic processes used to confirm monkeypox infections, emphasising the role of laboratory testing in accurate diagnosis.
- **Treatment and Vaccination**: An overview of current treatment options and vaccination strategies, including the use of antiviral medications and the smallpox vaccine.
- **Self-care and Prevention**: Practical advice on how individuals and communities can protect themselves from monkeypox infection, focusing on hygiene, protective measures, and community education.
- **Outbreaks**: Case studies of recent monkeypox outbreaks, analysing the factors that led to these events and the lessons learned from the response efforts.
- **WHO Response**: A look at the World Health Organization's role in managing monkeypox outbreaks, including surveillance, risk assessment, and global coordination.
- **Patient's Guide to Mpox Treatment with TPOXX (Tecovirimat)**: Detailed guidance on the use of Tecovirimat, an antiviral medication approved for monkeypox treatment, including usage instructions, dosage, and potential side effects.
- **Mpox Monitoring and Risk Assessment for Persons Exposed in the Community**: Strategies for monitoring and assessing the risk of monkeypox in individuals exposed in community settings, providing a framework for effective public health interventions.

Raj Kishor Mahapatra's book serves as an invaluable resource for anyone looking to deepen their understanding of the monkeypox virus and its implications. Whether you are a healthcare professional seeking detailed information or a concerned individual looking for practical advice, this book offers the knowledge and tools needed to navigate the challenges posed by the MPOX virus.

KEY FACTS

1. **Zoonotic Disease**: Monkeypox is a viral zoonotic disease, meaning it can spread from animals to humans. It was first discovered in 1958 in laboratory monkeys, with the first human case recorded in 1970 in the Democratic Republic of Congo.
2. **Virus Family**: Monkeypox virus belongs to the Orthopoxvirus genus in the family Poxviridae, which also includes the variola virus (which causes smallpox), vaccinia virus (used in the smallpox vaccine), and cowpox virus.
3. **Geographic Distribution**: Historically, monkeypox has been endemic in Central and West African countries. However, recent outbreaks have occurred in non-endemic regions, raising global health concerns.
4. **Reservoir Hosts**: The exact reservoir of monkeypox remains unknown, but African rodents and non-human primates (like monkeys) are suspected to play a role in the transmission of the virus to humans.
5. **Transmission**: The virus can spread to humans through direct contact with the blood, bodily fluids, or cutaneous or mucosal lesions of infected animals. Human-to-human transmission can occur through respiratory droplets, direct contact with body fluids, or contact with contaminated materials like bedding.
6. **Incubation Period**: The incubation period for monkeypox is usually 6 to 13 days but can range from 5 to 21 days. This period refers to the time from initial infection to the onset of symptoms.

7. **Symptoms**: Initial symptoms include fever, headache, muscle aches, backache, swollen lymph nodes, chills, and exhaustion. A rash usually develops 1-3 days after the fever, beginning on the face and spreading to other parts of the body.
8. **Rash Progression**: The rash progresses through several stages before forming scabs: macules (flat lesions), papules (raised lesions), vesicles (fluid-filled lesions), pustules (pus-filled lesions), and then scabs.
9. **Mortality Rate**: The case fatality rate for monkeypox can vary but has been reported to be around 1-10% in Africa. The rate may be lower in non-endemic regions due to better access to healthcare.
10. **Diagnosis**: Laboratory tests, such as polymerase chain reaction (PCR), are essential for diagnosing monkeypox. Serological tests and virus isolation can also be used.
11. **Treatment**: There is no specific treatment for monkeypox, but antiviral drugs like tecovirimat (TPOXX) have been approved for use in some regions. Supportive care and symptomatic treatment are critical for patient recovery.
12. **Vaccination**: Vaccination against smallpox has been shown to provide cross-protection against monkeypox. Newer vaccines specifically for monkeypox are under development and have been used in outbreak control.
13. **Prevention**: Preventive measures include avoiding contact with animals that could harbour the virus, practising good hand hygiene, and using personal protective equipment when caring for infected patients.
14. **Recent Outbreaks**: Notable recent outbreaks have occurred in non-endemic regions, including the United States and parts of Europe, often linked to international travel or the importation of animals.
15. **WHO Involvement**: The World Health Organization (WHO) monitors monkeypox outbreaks, provides guidance for managing cases, and supports countries

in strengthening their surveillance and response capacities.
16. **Public Health Challenge**: Monkeypox poses a significant public health challenge due to its potential for widespread outbreaks, the need for rapid response and containment measures, and the importance of international cooperation.

Understanding these key facts about monkeypox is essential for effective prevention, diagnosis, and treatment, as well as for implementing appropriate public health measures to control the spread of the virus.

-

OVERVIEW

Monkeypox is a viral zoonotic disease caused by the monkeypox virus, a member of the Orthopoxvirus genus in the family Poxviridae. The disease was first identified in 1958 when outbreaks occurred in colonies of monkeys kept for research, hence the name "monkeypox." The first human case of monkeypox was reported in 1970 in the Democratic Republic of Congo during intensified efforts to eliminate smallpox. Since then, monkeypox has been reported in several Central and West African countries, becoming endemic in these regions.

Historical Context

Monkeypox emerged as a notable pathogen in the 20th century, especially after the eradication of smallpox in 1980, which led to the cessation of smallpox vaccination programs. This vaccination also provided cross-protection against monkeypox. The cessation of this program has contributed to the increasing susceptibility of the human population to monkeypox infection.

Epidemiology

Monkeypox is endemic to Central and West Africa, particularly in countries like the Democratic Republic of Congo, Nigeria, and Cameroon. However, recent years have seen outbreaks in non-endemic regions, including Europe and North America. These outbreaks are often linked to international travel or the importation of infected animals, highlighting the global nature of the threat posed by monkeypox.

Virus Reservoir and Hosts

The natural reservoir of the monkeypox virus remains unknown, but African rodents, including squirrels and rats, are suspected to play a significant role in maintaining the virus in nature. Non-human primates, such as monkeys, can also be infected and can transmit the virus to humans. Understanding the animal reservoirs is crucial for implementing effective control measures.

Transmission

Monkeypox virus transmission can occur through various routes:

- **Animal-to-Human Transmission**: Direct contact with the blood, bodily fluids, or cutaneous or mucosal lesions of infected animals. Eating undercooked meat and other animal products of infected animals is a possible risk factor.
- **Human-to-Human Transmission**: Close contact with respiratory secretions, skin lesions of an infected person, or recently contaminated objects. Transmission via respiratory droplets usually requires prolonged face-to-face contact, which puts healthcare workers, household members, and other close contacts of active cases at greater risk.

Clinical Features

Monkeypox presents with a prodromal phase characterised by fever, intense headache, muscle aches, back pain, low energy, and swollen lymph nodes. This is followed by a rash that typically starts on the face and spreads to other parts of the body, including palms of the hands and soles of the feet. The rash evolves sequentially from macules to papules, vesicles, pustules, and scabs. The severity of the disease can vary widely, with some cases being mild while others can be severe or even fatal.

Diagnosis and Treatment

Diagnosis of monkeypox is confirmed through laboratory tests, primarily polymerase chain reaction (PCR) testing, which is the gold standard due to its accuracy. Other methods include serological tests and virus isolation. There is no specific treatment for monkeypox, but antiviral agents like tecovirimat (TPOXX) have been approved in some regions to treat monkeypox.

Management mainly involves supportive care to alleviate symptoms and prevent complications.

Prevention

Preventive measures include avoiding contact with animals that could harbour the virus, practising good hand hygiene, and using protective equipment when caring for infected patients. Vaccination against smallpox has been found to provide cross-protection against monkeypox. Newer vaccines specifically targeting monkeypox are being developed and have been used in recent outbreak responses.

Public Health Response

The recent spread of monkeypox to non-endemic regions has prompted public health authorities worldwide to strengthen surveillance, improve diagnostic capacities, and develop strategic vaccination campaigns. The World Health Organization (WHO) plays a critical role in coordinating global efforts to monitor and respond to monkeypox outbreaks.

Global Impact

The increasing frequency and geographic spread of monkeypox outbreaks pose a significant public health challenge. International collaboration is essential to address these outbreaks through timely detection, effective response, and long-term strategies to prevent future occurrences. Understanding the dynamics of monkeypox transmission and implementing comprehensive control measures are vital steps toward mitigating the impact of this re-emerging infectious disease.

This book aims to provide a thorough understanding of monkeypox, its transmission dynamics, clinical management, and prevention strategies, serving as a valuable resource for healthcare professionals, policymakers, and the general public. By enhancing our knowledge and response capabilities, we can better manage and control the spread of monkeypox, safeguarding global health.

TRANSMISSION

Understanding the transmission mechanisms of the MPOX (monkeypox) virus is crucial for implementing effective prevention and control measures. The monkeypox virus can spread from animals to humans (zoonotic transmission) and between humans (human-to-human transmission). The virus's transmission pathways highlight the importance of maintaining vigilance in both endemic and non-endemic regions to control its spread.

Zoonotic Transmission

Monkeypox is primarily a zoonotic disease, meaning it can be transmitted from animals to humans. The following points detail the zoonotic transmission routes:

1. **Animal Reservoirs**: While the exact natural reservoir of the monkeypox virus remains unidentified, African rodents, including rope squirrels, tree squirrels, Gambian pouched rats, and dormice, are considered potential reservoirs. Non-human primates, such as monkeys, can also be infected and serve as sources of transmission to humans.
2. **Direct Contact**: Humans can acquire the monkeypox virus through direct contact with the blood, bodily fluids, or cutaneous or mucosal lesions of infected animals. Handling infected animals without appropriate protective measures increases the risk of zoonotic transmission.
3. **Consumption of Infected Meat**: Consuming undercooked meat or other products from infected

animals poses a risk of transmission. This route of transmission underscores the importance of safe food handling practices, especially in regions where monkeypox is endemic.

Human-to-Human Transmission

Once the monkeypox virus infects a human, it can spread to other individuals through several mechanisms:

1. **Respiratory Droplets**: Human-to-human transmission can occur through large respiratory droplets. This usually requires prolonged face-to-face contact, making healthcare workers, household members, and other close contacts of active cases particularly vulnerable. Activities such as talking, coughing, or sneezing can facilitate the spread of respiratory droplets containing the virus.
2. **Direct Contact with Lesions**: Direct physical contact with the skin lesions or scabs of an infected person can transmit the virus. The virus can enter the body through broken skin, mucous membranes, or respiratory tract.
3. **Contaminated Objects**: The monkeypox virus can survive on surfaces and objects, such as bedding, clothing, and towels, that have been in contact with an infected person's bodily fluids or skin lesions. Handling these contaminated materials can lead to infection if proper hygiene and disinfection practices are not followed.
4. **Vertical Transmission**: There is potential for vertical transmission (from mother to foetus) during pregnancy, which can lead to congenital monkeypox. However, the frequency and impact of vertical transmission are still under investigation.

Factors Influencing Transmission

Several factors can influence the transmission dynamics of the monkeypox virus:

1. **Viral Load**: The amount of virus present in an infected person's bodily fluids and lesions can affect the likelihood of transmission. Higher viral loads may increase the risk of spreading the virus to others.
2. **Duration of Contact**: Prolonged exposure to an infected individual or contaminated environment increases the risk of transmission. This is particularly relevant in household settings and healthcare facilities.
3. **Immune Status**: Individuals with compromised immune systems or those who have not been vaccinated against smallpox may be more susceptible to infection and severe disease.
4. **Environmental Conditions**: The virus's survival on surfaces and in the environment can be influenced by factors such as temperature, humidity, and the presence of organic material. Proper cleaning and disinfection are essential to reduce the risk of environmental transmission.

Preventive Measures

To mitigate the transmission of the monkeypox virus, several preventive measures can be implemented:

1. **Avoid Contact with Wild Animals**: In endemic regions, minimising contact with wild animals, especially those that may harbour the virus, is crucial. This includes avoiding hunting, handling, and consuming wild game.
2. **Personal Protective Equipment (PPE)**: Healthcare workers and caregivers should use appropriate PPE, including masks, gloves, and gowns, when caring for infected individuals. This reduces the risk of respiratory and contact transmission.
3. **Hand Hygiene**: Regular handwashing with soap and water or using alcohol-based hand sanitizers can help prevent the spread of the virus. Hand hygiene

is especially important after contact with infected individuals or contaminated objects.
4. **Safe Handling of Infected Materials**: Proper disposal and disinfection of materials contaminated with bodily fluids or skin lesions are essential to prevent the virus from spreading. This includes bedding, clothing, and medical equipment.
5. **Vaccination**: Vaccination against smallpox provides cross-protection against monkeypox. Newer vaccines specifically targeting monkeypox are being developed and deployed in outbreak settings to control the spread.
6. **Public Health Surveillance**: Robust surveillance systems can detect and respond to monkeypox cases promptly. Early identification and isolation of cases, contact tracing, and quarantine measures are critical for controlling outbreaks.

Understanding the transmission pathways of the monkeypox virus and implementing effective preventive measures are essential steps in controlling the spread of this emerging infectious disease. By adopting a comprehensive approach to prevention, surveillance, and response, public health authorities can mitigate the impact of monkeypox and protect global health.

SIGNS AND SYMPTOMS

The signs and symptoms of monkeypox (MPOX) are similar to those of smallpox but generally milder. The clinical course of monkeypox can be divided into two periods: the invasion period and the skin eruption period.

Invasion Period

The invasion period lasts between 0-5 days and is characterised by several non-specific symptoms:

1. **Fever**: One of the earliest and most common symptoms. The fever is typically high, reaching 38-40°C (100.4-104°F).
2. **Severe Headache**: Intense headaches often accompany the fever.
3. **Muscle Aches (Myalgia)**: Patients may experience significant muscle pain.
4. **Back Pain**: Backache is a frequent complaint during the early stages.
5. **Swollen Lymph Nodes (Lymphadenopathy)**: Unlike smallpox, monkeypox infection causes noticeable swelling of the lymph nodes. This can occur in the neck, armpits, and groyne and is a key distinguishing feature.
6. **Chills and Exhaustion**: Patients often feel extremely tired and may experience chills.

Skin Eruption Period

The skin eruption period begins within 1-3 days after the

appearance of fever. The rash typically follows a specific progression through several stages:

1. **Macules**: Flat, discoloured spots on the skin, usually starting on the face and then spreading to other parts of the body, including the palms of the hands and soles of the feet.
2. **Papules**: Raised bumps that develop from macules.
3. **Vesicles**: Fluid-filled blisters that form from papules.
4. **Pustules**: Pus-filled lesions that develop from vesicles. These are often deep-seated, round, and firm to the touch.
5. **Scabs**: The pustules eventually crust over and form scabs. These scabs will fall off after about 10 days, leaving pitted scars.

The rash tends to be more concentrated on the face and extremities rather than on the trunk. Lesions can also appear on the mucous membranes of the mouth, genitals, and eyes. The number of lesions can vary from a few to several thousand, and they are typically at the same stage of development in a particular body area.

Other Symptoms

1. **Respiratory Symptoms**: In some cases, patients may experience sore throat, nasal congestion, or cough.
2. **Gastrointestinal Symptoms**: Nausea, vomiting, and diarrhoea can occur in some patients.
3. **Conjunctivitis**: Eye infections and inflammation can occur if the virus spreads to the eyes.

Severity and Duration

The severity of monkeypox can vary widely. While many cases are mild and self-limiting, some can be severe, especially in individuals with compromised immune systems or underlying health conditions. The disease typically lasts for 2-4 weeks from the onset of symptoms to the resolution of the rash and other symptoms.

Complications

Complications of monkeypox can include secondary bacterial infections of the skin lesions, respiratory distress, pneumonia, sepsis, encephalitis, and eye infections, which can lead to vision loss. Severe cases can be fatal, with the case fatality rate varying between 1-10% in African outbreaks, depending on the strain and the patient's health status.

Differentiating from Similar Diseases

Monkeypox can be mistaken for other rash illnesses such as chickenpox, measles, bacterial skin infections, scabies, syphilis, and medication-associated allergies. However, the presence of lymphadenopathy, the synchronous progression of lesions, and the overall clinical picture help differentiate monkeypox from these conditions.

Understanding the signs and symptoms of monkeypox is crucial for early detection, diagnosis, and isolation of cases to prevent the spread of the virus. Healthcare providers should be vigilant, especially in regions with reported cases or where the virus is endemic.

DIAGNOSIS

Diagnosing monkeypox (MPOX) involves a combination of clinical evaluation, patient history, and laboratory testing. Due to its similarity to other pox-like diseases, a thorough and accurate diagnosis is essential for appropriate management and containment of the disease.

Clinical Evaluation

1. **Symptom Assessment**: Healthcare providers begin by evaluating the patient's symptoms, focusing on key signs such as fever, headache, muscle aches, back pain, and the characteristic rash. The presence of swollen lymph nodes (lymphadenopathy) is particularly indicative, as it helps distinguish monkeypox from smallpox.
2. **Rash Examination**: The progression of the rash from macules to papules, vesicles, pustules, and eventually scabs is a critical diagnostic feature. The distribution of lesions, particularly on the face, palms, and soles, along with the synchronous development of the rash in specific areas, provides important clues.
3. **Patient History**: A detailed history is crucial, including recent travel to endemic areas, contact with animals (especially rodents or non-human primates), and exposure to individuals with similar symptoms. Identifying potential exposure sources helps narrow down the diagnosis.

Laboratory Testing

Laboratory confirmation is essential for a definitive diagnosis of monkeypox. The following tests are commonly used:

1. **Polymerase Chain Reaction (PCR)**: PCR is the gold standard for monkeypox diagnosis due to its high sensitivity and specificity. Samples are typically taken from skin lesions (fluid from vesicles and pustules or crusts from scabs). PCR can detect viral DNA, confirming the presence of the monkeypox virus.
2. **Serological Tests**: These tests detect antibodies against the monkeypox virus in the patient's blood. While useful, serological tests are less specific than PCR and are often used in conjunction with other diagnostic methods. They can help determine if a person has been previously exposed to the virus.
3. **Virus Isolation**: This involves culturing the virus from clinical specimens, such as lesion samples, in a laboratory setting. Although highly specific, this method is time-consuming and requires specialised facilities, making it less commonly used in routine diagnostics.
4. **Histopathology**: Microscopic examination of tissue samples from skin lesions can provide additional diagnostic information. Characteristic findings include eosinophilic cytoplasmic inclusions and necrosis of the epidermis.
5. **Electron Microscopy**: This technique allows for the visualisation of viral particles in clinical samples. While it provides a definitive diagnosis, it is not widely available in most clinical settings.

Differential Diagnosis

Differentiating monkeypox from other similar diseases is crucial to avoid misdiagnosis. Conditions with similar clinical presentations include:

1. **Chickenpox (Varicella)**: Caused by the varicella-zoster virus, chickenpox presents with a similar vesicular rash. However, the absence of lymphadenopathy and the asynchronous progression of lesions (different stages of development) help distinguish it from monkeypox.
2. **Smallpox**: Although eradicated, smallpox shared several features with monkeypox. The key difference is that smallpox does not cause lymphadenopathy. Vaccination history also aids in differentiation.
3. **Measles**: Measles presents with fever, rash, and respiratory symptoms. The rash typically starts on the face and spreads downwards, but it lacks the vesicular and pustular stages seen in monkeypox.
4. **Bacterial Skin Infections**: Conditions like impetigo can mimic the pustular rash of monkeypox. Bacterial culture and sensitivity testing can help differentiate these infections.
5. **Syphilis**: Secondary syphilis can cause a generalised rash that may resemble monkeypox. Serological tests for syphilis aid in differentiation.

Reporting and Notification

Monkeypox is a notifiable disease in many countries. Healthcare providers must report suspected and confirmed cases to public health authorities. Prompt reporting facilitates contact tracing, outbreak investigation, and implementation of control measures.

Importance of Accurate Diagnosis

Accurate diagnosis of monkeypox is vital for several reasons:

1. **Patient Management**: Confirming the diagnosis ensures that patients receive appropriate care, including supportive treatment and antiviral therapy if indicated.
2. **Infection Control**: Identifying cases early allows for timely isolation of patients and implementation of infection control measures to prevent further spread.

3. **Public Health Response**: Accurate diagnosis supports public health surveillance and response efforts, helping to contain outbreaks and prevent wider transmission.
4. **Research and Understanding**: Confirmed cases contribute to the global understanding of monkeypox epidemiology, aiding in the development of better diagnostic tools, treatments, and vaccines.

In conclusion, the diagnosis of monkeypox involves a combination of clinical evaluation, patient history, and laboratory testing. Accurate and timely diagnosis is crucial for effective patient management, infection control, and public health response. Healthcare providers must remain vigilant and consider monkeypox in patients presenting with compatible symptoms, especially in the context of travel to endemic areas or known exposure to the virus.

TREATMENT AND VACCINATION

Treatment

Currently, there are no specific treatments for monkeypox virus infections. However, several therapeutic approaches can help manage and alleviate symptoms, prevent complications, and support recovery. These include supportive care, antiviral medications, and treatment of secondary infections.

1. **Supportive Care**:
   - **Hydration**: Ensuring adequate fluid intake to prevent dehydration, which can result from fever and reduced oral intake.
   - **Pain Management**: Administering analgesics like acetaminophen or ibuprofen to reduce fever and alleviate pain.
   - **Skin Care**: Keeping skin lesions clean and dry to prevent secondary bacterial infections. Applying antiseptic solutions to lesions may help.
   - **Nutritional Support**: Maintaining adequate nutrition to support the immune system during recovery.
2. **Antiviral Medications**:
   - **Tecovirimat (TPOXX)**: Tecovirimat is an antiviral medication approved by the US FDA for the treatment of smallpox, and it has shown efficacy against orthopoxviruses, including monkeypox. It works by inhibiting the activity of the viral protein, preventing virus replication.

- **Cidofovir**: This antiviral is also used to treat severe orthopoxvirus infections. It inhibits viral DNA synthesis. Due to potential renal toxicity, its use requires careful monitoring.
- **Brincidofovir**: A lipid conjugate of cidofovir, it has shown promise in treating orthopoxvirus infections with potentially less nephrotoxicity compared to cidofovir.

3. **Treating Secondary Infections**:
   - **Antibiotics**: If secondary bacterial infections occur, appropriate antibiotics should be administered. Skin lesions can become infected with bacteria, necessitating antibiotic treatment.
4. **Isolation and Infection Control**:
   - **Isolation**: Infected individuals should be isolated to prevent the spread of the virus. Healthcare workers should use appropriate personal protective equipment (PPE).
   - **Barrier Nursing Techniques**: Implementing strict infection control measures in healthcare settings to prevent transmission.

Vaccination

Vaccination plays a crucial role in preventing monkeypox infections and controlling outbreaks. The following vaccines are relevant in the context of monkeypox:

1. **Smallpox Vaccine**:
   - The smallpox vaccine provides cross-protection against monkeypox due to the genetic similarities between the smallpox virus (variola virus) and the monkeypox virus.
   - **First-Generation Smallpox Vaccines**: These vaccines, such as Dryvax, were highly effective in eradicating smallpox and provide immunity against monkeypox. However, due to adverse effects, they are not widely

used today.
2. **Second-Generation Smallpox Vaccines**:
   o   **ACAM2000**: This live, attenuated vaccine is derived from a clone of Dryvax. It has an improved safety profile compared to first-generation vaccines but still carries some risks of adverse effects. It is used primarily for specific populations, such as laboratory workers handling orthopoxviruses.
3. **Third-Generation Smallpox Vaccines**:
   o   **MVA-BN (Modified Vaccinia Ankara – Bavarian Nordic)**: Also known as Imvamune or Imvanex, this vaccine is a highly attenuated, non-replicating vaccine. It has been approved in some countries for immunisation against smallpox and monkeypox. It is considered safer, especially for individuals with weakened immune systems.

Vaccination Strategies

1. **Pre-Exposure Vaccination**:
   o   Administering vaccines to individuals at high risk of exposure, such as healthcare workers, laboratory personnel, and animal handlers in endemic regions. This proactive approach helps protect those most likely to encounter the virus.
2. **Post-Exposure Prophylaxis (PEP)**:
   o   Vaccination within 4 days of exposure to the monkeypox virus can prevent the onset of the disease. Vaccination between 4-14 days after exposure can reduce the severity of the disease. This strategy is critical for controlling outbreaks and protecting close contacts of confirmed cases.
3. **Ring Vaccination**:
   o   This strategy involves vaccinating the contacts of confirmed cases and their contacts (a "ring" of individuals) to create a buffer of immune individuals, thus preventing further transmission.

Ring vaccination was successfully used in the eradication of smallpox and can be effective in controlling monkeypox outbreaks.

Public Health Considerations

1. **Vaccine Supply and Distribution:**
   - Ensuring an adequate supply of vaccines and an efficient distribution system is vital for effective outbreak control. Coordination between public health authorities and vaccine manufacturers is essential.
2. **Education and Awareness:**
   - Public health campaigns should educate communities about the benefits of vaccination, the signs and symptoms of monkeypox, and preventive measures to reduce the risk of infection.
3. **Surveillance and Monitoring:**
   - Robust surveillance systems are necessary to detect and respond to monkeypox cases promptly. Monitoring vaccine coverage and efficacy helps inform public health strategies and improve outcomes.

Challenges and Future Directions

1. **Vaccine Hesitancy:**
   - Addressing vaccine hesitancy through transparent communication, addressing concerns, and providing evidence-based information is crucial for achieving high vaccination coverage.
2. **Research and Development:**
   - Continued research into the development of more effective and safer vaccines and antiviral treatments is essential. Investment in understanding the monkeypox virus and its transmission dynamics can lead to better prevention and control measures.
3. **Global Cooperation:**
   - International collaboration is necessary to control monkeypox, especially in regions where the

virus is endemic. Sharing resources, knowledge, and best practices can help manage outbreaks and prevent global spread.

In conclusion, while there are no specific treatments for monkeypox, supportive care, antiviral medications, and the management of secondary infections can help patients recover. Vaccination remains a cornerstone of monkeypox prevention and control, with strategies like pre-exposure vaccination, post-exposure prophylaxis, and ring vaccination playing vital roles. Public health efforts, education, and global cooperation are essential for managing and mitigating the impact of monkeypox.

SELF-CARE AND PREVENTION

Effective self-care and prevention strategies are crucial for controlling the spread of monkeypox (MPOX) and minimising its impact on individuals and communities. By understanding and implementing these measures, people can protect themselves and others from infection.

Self-care

1. **Isolation and Rest**:
   - If diagnosed with monkeypox or if symptoms suggestive of monkeypox are present, it is essential to stay at home and avoid close contact with others. Isolation helps prevent the spread of the virus.
   - Adequate rest is crucial to support the immune system in fighting the infection. Patients should ensure they get enough sleep and avoid strenuous activities.
2. **Hydration and Nutrition**:
   - Drinking plenty of fluids, such as water, herbal teas, and clear broths, helps prevent dehydration, which can result from fever and reduced fluid intake.
   - Maintaining a balanced diet rich in vitamins and minerals supports overall health and immune function. Consuming fruits, vegetables, lean proteins, and whole grains can aid in recovery.
3. **Skin Care**:
   - Keeping skin lesions clean and dry is vital to prevent secondary bacterial infections. Using antiseptic

solutions to cleanse the lesions can be beneficial.
- Avoid scratching or picking at the lesions to prevent scarring and further infection. Covering lesions with sterile dressings can help protect them.

4. **Symptom Management**:
   - Over-the-counter medications, such as acetaminophen or ibuprofen, can help reduce fever and alleviate pain.
   - Antihistamines may be used to relieve itching associated with skin lesions.

5. **Mental Health Support**:
   - Experiencing a monkeypox infection can be stressful and anxiety-inducing. Seeking support from friends, family, or mental health professionals can help manage stress and emotional well-being.

Prevention

Preventing monkeypox involves a combination of personal precautions, public health measures, and community awareness. Here are key strategies for preventing the spread of monkeypox:

1. **Avoid Contact with Infected Individuals**:
   - Avoid close physical contact with individuals who have symptoms of monkeypox, especially those with visible skin lesions.
   - Refrain from touching bedding, clothing, and other personal items used by an infected person.

2. **Hygiene Practices**:
   - Regular handwashing with soap and water is one of the most effective ways to prevent the spread of infectious diseases. Use hand sanitizer with at least 60% alcohol if soap and water are not available.
   - Practising good respiratory hygiene, such as covering the mouth and nose with a tissue or elbow when coughing or sneezing, can reduce the spread of respiratory droplets.

3. **Safe Animal Handling**:

- Avoid contact with wild animals, especially rodents and non-human primates, as they can be reservoirs for the monkeypox virus.
- When handling animals, particularly in endemic regions, use protective equipment and follow proper sanitation protocols.

4. **Vaccination**:
- Vaccination is a critical tool in preventing monkeypox. Individuals at high risk, such as healthcare workers, laboratory personnel, and animal handlers, should receive the smallpox vaccine, which provides cross-protection against monkeypox.
- During outbreaks, ring vaccination strategies can be employed to vaccinate contacts of confirmed cases and their contacts, creating a buffer of immune individuals.

5. **Travel Precautions**:
- Travellers to regions where monkeypox is endemic should take precautions, such as avoiding contact with animals that could harbour the virus and practising good hygiene.
- Stay informed about travel advisories and guidelines from health authorities.

6. **Public Health Measures**:
- Public health authorities play a crucial role in preventing and controlling monkeypox outbreaks. Measures include surveillance, contact tracing, and the implementation of quarantine and isolation protocols.
- Educating the public about monkeypox, its symptoms, and prevention strategies is essential for raising awareness and promoting preventive behaviours.

Community Awareness and Education

1. **Community Engagement**:
- Engaging with communities through awareness campaigns and educational programs helps disseminate information about monkeypox and

preventive measures.
- Collaboration with community leaders, healthcare providers, and organisations can enhance the reach and effectiveness of these efforts.

2. **Health Education**:
- Providing accurate and up-to-date information about monkeypox, including its transmission, symptoms, and prevention, empowers individuals to take proactive steps to protect themselves and their communities.
- Educational materials, such as brochures, posters, and online resources, can be distributed in multiple languages to ensure accessibility.

Role of Healthcare Providers

1. **Early Detection and Diagnosis**:
- Healthcare providers should be vigilant in recognizing the signs and symptoms of monkeypox, especially in patients with recent travel to endemic areas or contact with potential sources of infection.
- Prompt diagnosis and reporting of suspected cases to public health authorities are crucial for controlling the spread.

2. **Patient Counseling and Support**:
- Educating patients about self-care measures and the importance of isolation during the infectious period helps prevent transmission.
- Providing support and resources for managing symptoms and accessing healthcare services is essential for patient care.

Global Cooperation and Research

1. **International Collaboration**:
- Cooperation between countries and international organisations, such as the World Health Organization (WHO), is vital for monitoring and responding to

monkeypox outbreaks.
- Sharing data, resources, and best practices enhances global efforts to prevent and control the disease.

2. **Research and Development**:
   - Ongoing research into monkeypox, its transmission dynamics, and effective treatments and vaccines is essential for improving prevention and management strategies.
   - Investing in the development of safer and more effective vaccines and antiviral therapies can significantly impact the control of monkeypox.

In conclusion, self-care and prevention strategies are fundamental in managing and mitigating the spread of monkeypox. By practising good hygiene, avoiding contact with infected individuals and animals, and supporting public health measures, individuals can protect themselves and contribute to the broader effort to control monkeypox outbreaks. Community awareness, education, and global cooperation are key components of a comprehensive approach to preventing and managing this emerging infectious disease.

OUTBREAKS

Monkeypox outbreaks have occurred sporadically in various parts of the world, particularly in Central and West Africa. Understanding the history, dynamics, and responses to these outbreaks provides valuable insights into managing and controlling the disease.

Historical Outbreaks

1. **Early Cases**:
   - **1970**: The first recognized human case of monkeypox was reported in the Democratic Republic of the Congo (formerly Zaire). The outbreak was identified in a 9-month-old boy in a rural area, marking the beginning of awareness of this zoonotic disease in humans.
   - **1970s-1980s**: Subsequent outbreaks were reported in various countries in Central and West Africa. These early outbreaks were generally small and localised, with limited international attention.
2. **1990s-2000s**:
   - **1996-1997**: A significant outbreak occurred in the Democratic Republic of the Congo, affecting hundreds of people. The outbreak highlighted the potential for monkeypox to cause substantial morbidity in regions with limited healthcare resources.
   - **2003**: The first known outbreak of monkeypox outside Africa occurred in the United States. The outbreak was traced to imported pet prairie dogs, which had been in contact with infected rodents from Africa. The outbreak resulted in 47 confirmed cases across several

states.

Recent Outbreaks

1. **2017-2018**:
   - **Nigeria**: An outbreak in Nigeria began in September 2017 and continued into 2018. It was the largest outbreak in Nigeria since the 1970s, with over 200 suspected cases reported. The outbreak involved multiple states and highlighted the need for enhanced surveillance and response capabilities.
2. **2018-2019**:
   - **Democratic Republic of the Congo**: The DRC experienced a significant outbreak with over 3,000 cases reported. The outbreak affected several provinces and demonstrated the challenges of controlling monkeypox in conflict-affected areas with limited healthcare infrastructure.
3. **2022-2023**:
   - **Global Outbreak**: A notable global outbreak of monkeypox began in mid-2022, with cases reported in countries outside of Africa for the first time on a larger scale. This outbreak involved numerous countries across different continents, with significant transmission occurring in Europe and the Americas. The outbreak was characterised by a higher number of cases in urban settings and among men who have sex with men (MSM), leading to increased awareness and response efforts.

Outbreak Dynamics

1. **Transmission Patterns**:
   - Monkeypox outbreaks often follow a pattern of initial cases in rural or peri-urban areas, with transmission spreading to urban centres over time. In endemic regions, the virus may persist in animal reservoirs, contributing to recurring outbreaks.

- In recent global outbreaks, transmission has occurred in diverse settings, including crowded urban areas and among populations with close social networks.

2. **Geographic Spread**:
   - Outbreaks have typically been localised to specific regions or countries. However, the recent global outbreak demonstrated the ability of monkeypox to spread internationally, facilitated by travel and interconnected communities.

3. **Impact on Public Health**:
   - Outbreaks place significant strain on public health systems, especially in regions with limited resources. Challenges include early detection, rapid response, and the need for adequate healthcare facilities and trained personnel.
   - Economic and social impacts include healthcare costs, loss of productivity, and disruption of daily life, particularly in affected communities.

Response Strategies

1. **Surveillance and Detection**:
   - Active surveillance is crucial for early detection of monkeypox cases. Health authorities monitor for cases of febrile rash illnesses, particularly in areas with known outbreaks or high-risk populations.
   - Laboratory testing is used to confirm cases and identify potential outbreaks. Prompt identification of cases enables timely implementation of control measures.

2. **Containment Measures**:
   - **Isolation**: Infected individuals are isolated to prevent further transmission. This includes home isolation or hospitalisation, depending on the severity of the illness.
   - **Contact Tracing**: Identifying and monitoring individuals who have been in contact with confirmed cases helps prevent the spread of the virus. Contacts

may be advised to quarantine and monitor for symptoms.
3. **Vaccination**:
   o Ring vaccination, targeting contacts of confirmed cases and their contacts, is used to create a buffer of immune individuals and prevent further spread.
   o Vaccination strategies vary depending on the outbreak's scale and location. In large-scale outbreaks, mass vaccination campaigns may be implemented.
4. **Public Health Communication**:
   o Educating the public about monkeypox, its symptoms, and preventive measures is essential for reducing stigma and promoting safe practices.
   o Health authorities provide regular updates on outbreak status, prevention measures, and vaccination availability.
5. **International Collaboration**:
   o Global cooperation and information sharing are critical for managing outbreaks. Organisations such as the World Health Organization (WHO) coordinate international response efforts and provide technical assistance.
   o Collaborative research efforts aim to improve understanding of monkeypox transmission, develop new vaccines and treatments, and enhance outbreak preparedness and response.

Lessons Learned

1. **Strengthening Surveillance Systems**:
   o Enhancing surveillance systems in endemic regions and improving global monitoring capabilities are essential for early detection and rapid response to outbreaks.
2. **Improving Healthcare Infrastructure**:
   o Investing in healthcare infrastructure, including laboratory capacity and healthcare worker

training, helps strengthen response efforts and manage outbreaks effectively.
3. **Enhancing Community Engagement**:
   o   Engaging communities in prevention and response efforts helps build trust and encourages adherence to public health measures. Community involvement is crucial for effective outbreak management.
4. **Advancing Research and Development**:
   o   Ongoing research into monkeypox epidemiology, vaccines, and treatments is necessary to improve prevention and control strategies. Investment in research helps prepare for future outbreaks and enhances global health security.

In conclusion, monkeypox outbreaks have demonstrated the importance of effective surveillance, containment, and response strategies. Historical and recent outbreaks underscore the need for continuous efforts to improve public health systems, enhance community engagement, and foster international collaboration. By learning from past experiences and implementing best practices, we can better manage and control monkeypox outbreaks and protect global health.

WHO RESPONSE

The World Health Organization (WHO) plays a central role in coordinating global efforts to manage and control monkeypox outbreaks. The organisation provides guidance, technical support, and resources to affected countries and works to enhance international collaboration and preparedness. Here is an overview of WHO's response to monkeypox:

1. Surveillance and Monitoring

- **Global Surveillance System**:
    - The WHO coordinates global surveillance efforts to monitor the spread of monkeypox and detect new cases. This involves collecting data from member states, analysing trends, and identifying potential outbreaks.
    - The WHO utilises its Global Outbreak Alert and Response Network (GOARN) to support real-time monitoring and response to emerging cases of monkeypox.
- **Data Collection and Reporting**:
    - WHO collects and disseminates data on monkeypox cases, including epidemiological information, case counts, and geographical distribution. This information helps track the progress of outbreaks and guide response efforts.
    - Member states are encouraged to report cases and outbreaks to WHO promptly. Timely reporting ensures that appropriate support and resources are mobilised.

2. Technical Guidance and Support

- **Guidelines and Recommendations**:
  - WHO provides technical guidelines and recommendations for managing monkeypox outbreaks. These include guidance on case detection, diagnosis, treatment, and infection control measures.
  - The organisation issues interim guidelines and updates based on the evolving understanding of the virus and outbreak dynamics.
- **Capacity Building**:
  - WHO supports capacity-building initiatives to strengthen healthcare systems in affected countries. This includes training healthcare workers, enhancing laboratory capabilities, and improving diagnostic and treatment facilities.
  - The organisation also provides technical assistance to help countries develop and implement effective outbreak response plans.

3. **Outbreak Response Coordination**

- **Emergency Response Teams**:
  - WHO deploys emergency response teams to support affected countries during outbreaks. These teams include experts in epidemiology, virology, and public health who provide on-the-ground assistance and coordination.
  - The organisation coordinates with national health authorities, non-governmental organisations (NGOs), and other international partners to ensure a comprehensive response.
- **Resource Mobilisation**:
  - WHO works to mobilise resources, including financial support, medical supplies, and vaccines, to assist countries in managing outbreaks. The organisation collaborates with donors, governments, and partners to secure and distribute necessary resources.

- o   In the event of a major outbreak, WHO may establish emergency funds to support rapid response efforts and address urgent needs.

4. Research and Development

- **Supporting Research Initiatives:**
  - o   WHO promotes and supports research into monkeypox to improve understanding of the virus, its transmission, and effective control measures. This includes funding research projects, coordinating studies, and sharing research findings.
  - o   The organisation collaborates with research institutions, universities, and pharmaceutical companies to advance the development of vaccines and treatments for monkeypox.
- **Innovation and Knowledge Sharing:**
  - o   WHO facilitates knowledge sharing among researchers, healthcare providers, and public health officials. This includes organising conferences, webinars, and workshops to disseminate information and best practices.
  - o   The organisation encourages innovation in surveillance, diagnostics, and treatment to enhance outbreak preparedness and response.

5. Public Health Communication

- **Information Dissemination:**
  - o   WHO provides timely and accurate information about monkeypox to the public, healthcare professionals, and policymakers. This includes issuing fact sheets, updates, and health alerts through various communication channels.
  - o   The organisation works to counter misinformation and provide clear guidance on prevention, symptoms, and treatment.
- **Awareness Campaigns:**

- WHO conducts awareness campaigns to educate communities about monkeypox and promote preventive measures. These campaigns aim to increase public understanding and encourage adherence to health recommendations.
    - The organisation collaborates with local and international media to reach a wide audience and ensure that accurate information is available.

6. International Collaboration

- **Coordination with Partners:**
    - WHO collaborates with international organisations, such as the Centers for Disease Control and Prevention (CDC), the European Centre for Disease Prevention and Control (ECDC), and Médecins Sans Frontières (MSF), to coordinate global response efforts.
    - The organisation works with regional and national health authorities to ensure a unified and effective response to outbreaks.
- **Global Health Security:**
    - WHO supports initiatives to strengthen global health security and preparedness for emerging infectious diseases. This includes promoting the International Health Regulations (IHR) and encouraging countries to enhance their surveillance and response capacities.
    - The organisation advocates for investment in health systems and infrastructure to improve resilience to future outbreaks.

7. Lessons Learned and Recommendations

- **Post-Outbreak Evaluation:**
    - After an outbreak, WHO conducts evaluations to assess the response efforts and identify lessons learned. These evaluations help refine strategies and improve future outbreak preparedness.
    - The organisation provides recommendations based on

the evaluation findings to enhance global and national response capacities.
- **Policy Development**:
  - WHO uses insights gained from outbreaks to inform policy development and strengthen international health regulations. This includes updating guidelines and protocols to reflect the latest evidence and best practices.

8. Future Preparedness

- **Strengthening Global Preparedness**:
  - WHO works to improve global preparedness for monkeypox and other emerging infectious diseases by supporting research, enhancing surveillance, and building response capacities.
  - The organisation advocates for a One Health approach that considers the interconnectedness of human, animal, and environmental health.

In summary, the World Health Organization plays a pivotal role in managing and controlling monkeypox outbreaks through surveillance, technical guidance, emergency response, research support, and public health communication. By coordinating international efforts and providing expertise and resources, WHO helps countries effectively respond to outbreaks and strengthen global health security.

PATIENT'S GUIDE TO MPOX TREATMENT WITH TPOXX (TECOVIRIMAT)

Introduction

Tecovirimat, sold under the brand name TPOXX, is an antiviral medication used to treat monkeypox (Mpox). This guide provides essential information on how to use TPOXX, including dosing, administration, potential side effects, and additional care tips. Always follow your healthcare provider's instructions and consult them with any concerns.

What is TPOXX?

TPOXX is an antiviral medication specifically designed to treat smallpox and other orthopoxvirus infections, including monkeypox. It works by inhibiting the virus's ability to replicate, helping reduce the severity and duration of the illness.

Indications for Use

- **Treatment of Mpox**: TPOXX is prescribed to treat monkeypox in adults and children. It is typically recommended for patients with moderate to severe cases or those at higher risk of complications.

Dosage and Administration

1. **Dosage**:
   - **Adults**: The standard dose for adults is 600 mg of TPOXX taken twice daily (every 12 hours) for 14 days.
   - **Children**: Dosage for children is based on body weight and must be determined by a healthcare provider. The typical dose is adjusted according to weight categories.
2. **Administration**:
   - TPOXX is taken orally in the form of a capsule or liquid suspension.
   - Capsules should be swallowed whole with a glass of water. Do not crush or chew the capsules.
   - If you are prescribed the liquid form, shake the bottle well before measuring the dose. Use the provided oral syringe to ensure accurate dosing.
3. **Missed Dose**:
   - If you miss a dose, take it as soon as you remember. If it is almost time for your next dose, skip the missed dose and continue with your regular schedule. Do not double the dose to make up for a missed one.

Precautions and Warnings

1. **Allergies and Sensitivities**:
   - Inform your healthcare provider if you have a known allergy to TPOXX or any of its components.
2. **Medical Conditions**:
   - Share your complete medical history with your healthcare provider, including any liver conditions, kidney problems, or other health issues.
3. **Pregnancy and Breastfeeding**:
   - TPOXX should be used during pregnancy only if the potential benefit justifies the potential risk to the foetus. Discuss with your healthcare provider if you are pregnant, plan to become pregnant, or are breastfeeding.
4. **Drug Interactions**:

- Inform your healthcare provider of all medications, including over-the-counter drugs and supplements, that you are currently taking. TPOXX may interact with other medications, affecting its efficacy or increasing side effects.

Side Effects

1. **Common Side Effects**:
   - **Gastrointestinal**: Nausea, vomiting, diarrhoea, and abdominal pain.
   - **General**: Headache, fatigue, and dizziness.
2. **Serious Side Effects**:
   - **Allergic Reactions**: Rash, itching, swelling of the face or throat, severe dizziness, or difficulty breathing.
   - **Liver Issues**: Yellowing of the skin or eyes (jaundice), dark urine, or persistent abdominal pain.
3. **Management of Side Effects**:
   - **Mild Side Effects**: These can often be managed with supportive care. Report any persistent or bothersome side effects to your healthcare provider.
   - **Severe Side Effects**: Seek immediate medical attention if you experience symptoms of a severe allergic reaction or significant liver issues.

Monitoring and Follow-Up

1. **Routine Check-Ups**:
   - Regular follow-up appointments with your healthcare provider are essential to monitor your response to treatment and adjust the dosage if necessary.
   - Your healthcare provider may perform blood tests or other evaluations to check for side effects and ensure the medication is effective.
2. **Report Concerns**:
   - Notify your healthcare provider if you experience any new or worsening symptoms. It is important to report any side effects promptly to address them

appropriately.

Self-Care and Lifestyle Adjustments

1. **Hydration and Nutrition**:
   - Maintain good hydration and eat a balanced diet to support overall health and recovery. Proper nutrition can help your body cope with the illness and side effects of medication.
2. **Rest and Recovery**:
   - Ensure adequate rest to aid in recovery. Avoid strenuous activities and focus on recuperating from the illness.
3. **Infection Control**:
   - Follow good hygiene practices to prevent the spread of monkeypox. This includes frequent handwashing, avoiding close contact with others, and covering any lesions.
4. **Support Systems**:
   - Seek support from family, friends, or mental health professionals if needed. Dealing with a serious illness can be stressful, and support can be beneficial.

Additional Tips

1. **Medication Adherence**:
   - Adhere strictly to the prescribed dosage and schedule. Missing doses or altering the dose can affect the treatment's effectiveness.
2. **Storage**:
   - Store TPOXX at room temperature, away from moisture and heat. Keep it out of reach of children.
3. **Travel and Activities**:
   - Consult with your healthcare provider before travelling or engaging in activities that might affect your treatment or health status.

Conclusion

TPOXX is an effective treatment for monkeypox when used as directed. Understanding how to properly take the medication, recognize potential side effects, and maintain good self-care practices will contribute to a successful treatment outcome. Always consult your healthcare provider with any questions or concerns about your treatment plan.

By following this guide and your healthcare provider's instructions, you can manage your monkeypox treatment effectively and support your recovery process.

MPOX MONITORING AND RISK ASSESSMENT FOR PERSONS EXPOSED IN THE COMMUNITY

Introduction

Monitoring and risk assessment for persons exposed to monkeypox (Mpox) in the community are crucial for preventing the spread of the disease and ensuring timely intervention. This guide provides comprehensive information on monitoring exposed individuals, assessing risk levels, and implementing appropriate public health measures.

1. Understanding Exposure Risk

1. **Types of Exposure**:
    - **Direct Contact**: Exposure through physical contact with an infected person's lesions, bodily fluids, or contaminated materials.
    - **Indirect Contact**: Exposure through contact with contaminated surfaces, clothing, or bedding.
    - **Close Proximity**: Prolonged face-to-face contact with an infected individual, particularly in settings where respiratory droplets can spread.
2. **Risk Factors**:

- **Type of Contact**: Direct and prolonged contact with infected individuals or their environment poses higher risk compared to brief, casual interactions.
- **Personal Protective Measures**: Individuals not using proper personal protective equipment (PPE) during exposure are at greater risk.
- **Health Status**: Individuals with compromised immune systems, underlying health conditions, or young children may be at higher risk of severe disease.

2. Monitoring Individuals for Symptoms

1. **Observation Period**:
   - Individuals exposed to monkeypox should be monitored for symptoms for a period of 21 days following exposure, as this is the maximum incubation period for the virus.
2. **Symptom Checklist**:
   - **Fever**: Monitor for elevated body temperature.
   - **Rash**: Watch for the development of a rash, particularly if it progresses from macules to papules and then to pustules.
   - **Respiratory Symptoms**: Note any cough, sore throat, or other respiratory issues.
   - **Other Symptoms**: Observe for muscle aches, headache, fatigue, and swollen lymph nodes.
3. **Daily Monitoring**:
   - Individuals should conduct daily self-checks for symptoms and maintain a symptom diary.
   - Healthcare providers may implement a daily phone or online check-in system for regular symptom updates and guidance.

3. Risk Assessment for Exposed Individuals

1. **Initial Assessment**:
   - **Exposure History**: Assess the nature and duration of exposure to determine risk level. Detailed information

about the type of contact and the use of protective measures is essential.
- **Health Assessment**: Evaluate the individual's current health status, including pre-existing conditions that may affect disease severity.

2. **Categorising Risk Levels**:
- **High Risk**: Direct, prolonged contact with an infected individual without protective measures. Individuals with compromised immune systems or pre-existing health conditions.
- **Moderate Risk**: Indirect contact or brief contact with an infected person, especially if PPE was not used.
- **Low Risk**: Casual or minimal contact with an infected individual, particularly if appropriate precautions were taken.

3. **Follow-Up Actions**:
- **High-Risk Individuals**: Implement stricter monitoring, including daily health checks and potential isolation if symptoms develop.
- **Moderate-Risk Individuals**: Regular symptom monitoring and adherence to preventive measures. Consider targeted testing if symptoms appear.
- **Low-Risk Individuals**: General monitoring and adherence to hygiene practices. No additional intervention is typically required unless symptoms develop.

4. Preventive Measures for Exposed Individuals

   1. **Personal Hygiene**:
   - **Hand Hygiene**: Wash hands frequently with soap and water or use hand sanitizer.
   - **Avoid Touching Face**: Refrain from touching the face, especially the eyes, nose, and mouth, with unwashed hands.
   2. **Isolation and Quarantine**:
   - **Self-Isolation**: Individuals exhibiting symptoms

should isolate themselves to prevent potential spread.
- **Quarantine**: Exposed individuals without symptoms may be advised to quarantine at home to minimise contact with others during the monitoring period.

3. **Protective Measures**:
   - **Use of PPE**: Wear masks, gloves, and other protective equipment as recommended, especially if in close contact with individuals at higher risk.
   - **Cleaning and Disinfection**: Regularly clean and disinfect surfaces and items that may have been contaminated.

4. **Health and Medical Advice**:
   - **Seek Medical Guidance**: Contact healthcare providers for advice if symptoms develop or if there are concerns about potential exposure.
   - **Vaccination**: Consider vaccination for individuals at high risk of exposure or severe disease, based on public health recommendations.

5. Reporting and Coordination

   1. **Reporting Procedures**:
      - **Notify Authorities**: Report cases and suspected cases of monkeypox to local public health authorities to facilitate monitoring and response efforts.
      - **Documentation**: Maintain accurate records of exposure events, symptom monitoring, and any interventions implemented.
   2. **Coordination with Health Services**:
      - **Local Health Departments**: Collaborate with local health departments to ensure coordination of response measures and access to resources.
      - **Healthcare Providers**: Work with healthcare providers to ensure timely testing, diagnosis, and treatment for exposed individuals.
   3. **Community Communication**:
      - **Public Awareness**: Provide accurate information

to the community about monkeypox, symptoms, and preventive measures.
- **Support Services**: Offer support services for individuals affected by monkeypox or those in quarantine, including mental health resources and assistance with daily needs.

6. Managing Potential Outbreaks

1. **Outbreak Detection**:
   - **Monitor Trends**: Observe for clusters of cases or increases in reported symptoms in the community that may indicate an outbreak.
   - **Investigate**: Conduct investigations to identify sources of exposure and implement containment measures as needed.
2. **Response Planning**:
   - **Emergency Plans**: Develop and implement emergency response plans for managing outbreaks, including resources for testing, treatment, and vaccination.
   - **Public Health Messaging**: Ensure clear and consistent communication with the public about outbreak status, preventive measures, and response actions.
3. **Evaluation and Improvement**:
   - **Assess Response**: Evaluate the effectiveness of monitoring and response efforts and make improvements based on lessons learned.
   - **Adapt Strategies**: Adjust monitoring and risk assessment strategies as needed based on evolving epidemiological data and public health recommendations.

Conclusion

Effective monitoring and risk assessment for persons exposed to monkeypox in the community are essential for controlling the spread of the disease and protecting public health. By following established procedures, implementing preventive measures, and maintaining clear communication, communities can better manage exposure risks and respond effectively to potential outbreaks. Always work closely with healthcare providers and public health authorities to ensure a coordinated and effective approach to managing monkeypox exposure.

THANK YOU MESSAGE

Dear Readers,

I want to extend my heartfelt gratitude to each of you for choosing to read *Mpox (Monkeypox) Virus: Why is it Spreading So Quickly?* Your interest and engagement with this book are truly appreciated.

Writing this book has been a journey of discovery and learning, and I hope that the information and insights shared within these pages have been both informative and valuable to you. My goal was to provide a comprehensive understanding of the Mpox virus, its transmission, and effective strategies for managing and preventing its spread. Your support and enthusiasm for this subject are vital in the collective effort to address and overcome the challenges posed by this virus.

Thank you for your commitment to learning and staying informed. Your curiosity and dedication play a crucial role in advancing public health and ensuring a safer, healthier future for us all.

Warm regards,

Raj Kishor Mahapatra

www.ingramcontent.com/pod-product-compliance
Lightning Source LLC
Chambersburg PA
CBHW030508220526
45464CB00006B/2712